KETO DIET COOKBOOK FOR WOMEN OVER 50

2021

50 Easy, Effective Low-Carb Recipes To Balance Hormones And Effortlessly Reach Your Weight Loss Goal.

GERALD COOPER

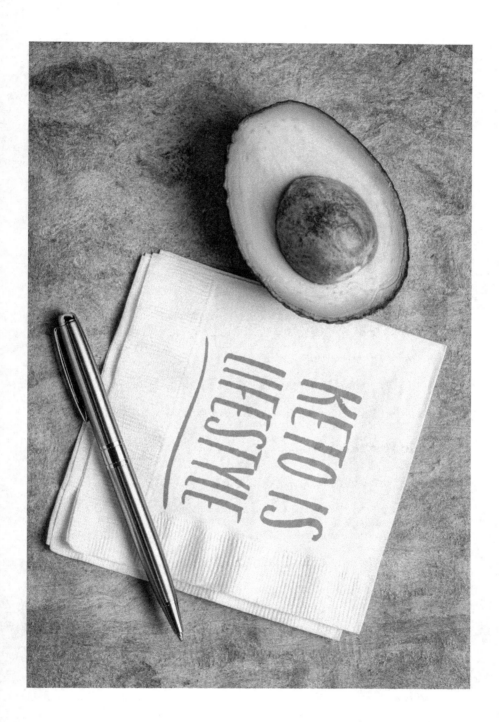

TABLE OF CONTENTS

Ketogenic Poultry Recipes 10

    Chicken and Salsa 10

    Creamy Turkey 12

    Duck and Zucchinis 14

    Chicken and Raspberries Salad 16

    Turkey and Spinach 18

    Turkey and Tomatoes 20

    Turkey and Cabbage Mix 22

    Chili Turkey and Broccoli 24

    Ground Turkey and Bell Peppers 26

    Chicken and Walnuts Salad 28

Ketogenic Meat Recipes 29

    Oregano Pork Chops 29

    Coconut Beef 31

    Beef, Tomato and Peppers 33

    Pork Meatballs 35

    Herbed Beef Mix 37

    Sage Beef 39

    Beef Casserole 41

    Thyme Beef and Leeks 43

    Coconut Pork and Celery 45

    Pork and Mushroom Meatloaf 47

Minty Beef *49*

Parsley Pork and Beef Meatballs *51*

Beef with Kale and Leeks *53*

Sesame Beef *55*

Marjoram Beef *57*

Ketogenic Vegetable Recipes **59**

Broccoli Cream *59*

Cauliflower and Tomatoes Mix *61*

Shallots and Kale Soup *63*

Hot Kale Pan *65*

Baked Broccoli *67*

Leeks Cream *69*

Fennel Soup *71*

Cauliflower and Green Beans *73*

Bok Choy Soup *75*

Cabbage Sauté *77*

Mustard Greens Sauté *79*

Bok Choy and Tomatoes *81*

Sesame Savoy Cabbage *83*

Chili Collard Greens *84*

Artichokes Soup *86*

Ketogenic Dessert Recipes **88**

Chocolate Pudding *88*

Coffee Cream *90*

Walnut Balls *91*

Vanilla Cream 93

Berry Cream 95

Cream Cheese Ramekins 97

Avocado Cream 98

Strawberry Stew 100

Coconut Muffins 102

Blueberries Mousse 104

RECIPE INDEX 108

MEASUREMENTS & CONVERSIONS 111

Ketogenic Poultry Recipes

Chicken and Salsa

Everyone will be impressed with this keto dish!

Preparation time: 10 minutes
Cooking time: 20 minutes
Servings: 4

Ingredients:
2 pounds chicken breasts, skinless, boneless and cubed
2 tablespoons olive oil
½ cup chicken stock
2 shallots, chopped
1 cup cherry tomatoes, halved
1 cup cucumber, cubed
1 cup black olives, pitted and sliced
¼ cup parsley, chopped
1 tablespoons lime juice

Directions:
Heat up a pan with the oil over medium heat, add the shallots, toss and cook for 2 minutes.

Add the chicken and brown for 5 minutes more. Add the tomatoes and the other ingredients, toss, cook over medium heat for 12-13 minutes more, divide into bowls and serve.

Nutrition: calories 230, fat 12, fiber 5.0, carbs 6.3, protein 20

Creamy Turkey

It's an extravagant dish but it's worth trying!

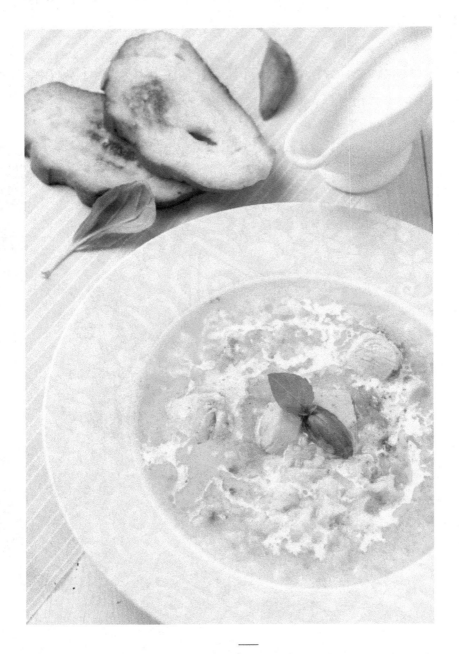

Preparation time: 10 minutes
Cooking time: 30 minutes
Servings: 4

Ingredients:

1 pound turkey breast, skinless, boneless and cubed
1 cup heavy cream
2 tablespoons olive oil
2 spring onions, chopped
2 leeks, chopped
A pinch of salt and black pepper
1 tablespoon cilantro, chopped

Directions:

Heat up a pan with the oil over medium heat, add the spring onions and the leeks and sauté for 2 minutes.
Add the meat and brown for 3 minutes more.
Add the rest of the ingredients, bring to a simmer and cook over medium heat for 25 minutes more, stirring often.
Divide the mix into bowls and serve.

Nutrition: calories 267, fat 5.6, fiber 0, carbs 6.0, protein 35

Duck and Zucchinis

If you are really hungry today then you should really try this recipe!

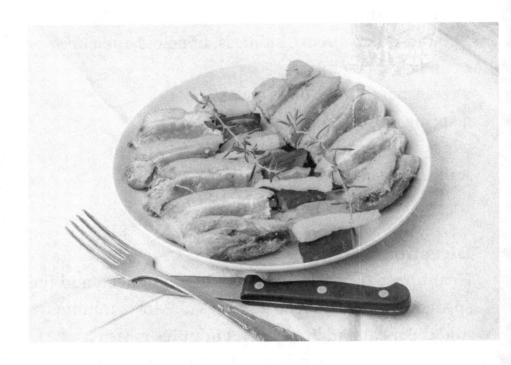

Preparation time: 10 minutes
Cooking time: 35 minutes
Servings: 4

Ingredients:
1 pound duck breasts, skinless, boneless and roughly cubed
2 zucchinis, sliced

1 tablespoon avocado oil
2 shallots, chopped
½ teaspoon chili powder
1 cup chicken stock
A pinch of salt and black pepper

Directions:
Heat up a pan with the oil over medium high heat, add the shallots, stir and sauté for 5 minutes.
Add the meat and the other ingredients, toss, bring to a simmer and cook over medium heat for 30 minutes.
Divide the mix into bowls and serve.

Nutrition: calories 450, fat 23, fiber 3, carbs 8.3, protein 50

Chicken and Raspberries Salad

It's a tasty salad and so easy to make!

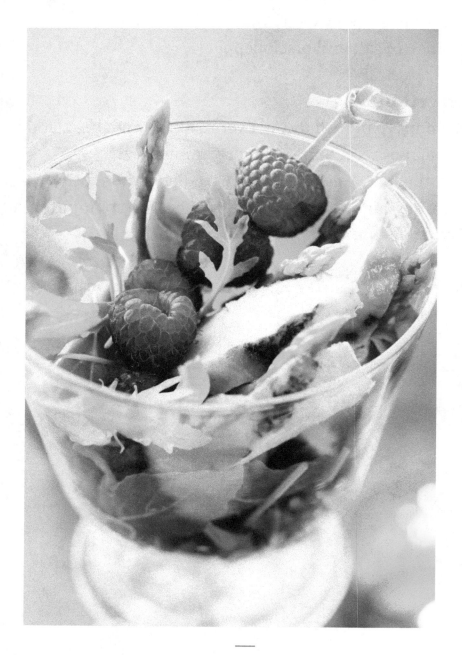

Preparation time: 10 minutes
Cooking time: 20 minutes
Servings: 4

Ingredients:
1 shallot, chopped
2 tablespoons olive oil
2 tablespoons balsamic vinegar
¼ cup chicken stock
1 cup raspberries
1 pound chicken breast, skinless, boneless and cut into strips
2 cups baby spinach
1 tablespoon cilantro, chopped

Directions:
Heat up a pan with the oil over medium heat, add the shallot and the chicken and brown for 5 minutes.
Add the remaining ingredients, toss, cook over medium heat for 15 minutes more, divide into bowls and serve.
Nutrition: calories 245, fat 13.40, fiber 4, carbs 5.6, protein 18

Turkey and Spinach

It's a great way to end your day!

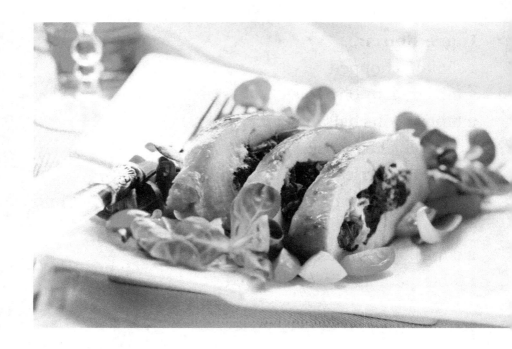

Preparation time: 10 minutes
Cooking time: 40 minutes
Servings: 6

Ingredients:
2 tablespoons olive oil
1 pound turkey breast, skinless, boneless and sliced
1 cup baby spinach
2 shallots, chopped

A pinch of salt and black pepper
Salt and black pepper to the taste
¼ teaspoon sweet paprika
¼ teaspoon garlic powder
1 tablespoon cilantro, chopped

Directions:
Heat up a pan with the oil over medium heat, add the meat and the shallots and brown for 5 minutes.
Add the spinach and the other ingredients, toss, bring to a simmer and cook over medium heat for 20 minutes.
Divide the mix in to bowls and serve.

Nutrition: calories 320, fat 23, fiber 8, carbs 6, protein 16

Turkey and Tomatoes

It's a very comforting and rich mix!

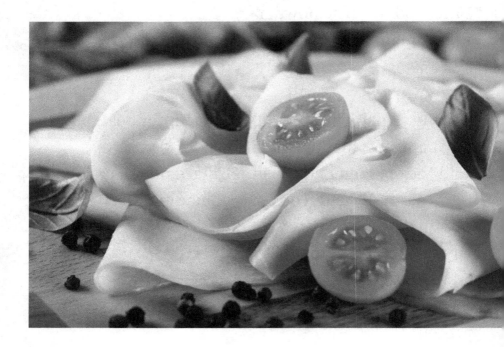

Preparation time: 10 minutes
Cooking time: 30 minutes
Servings: 4

Ingredients:
2 shallots, chopped
1 tablespoon ghee, melted
1 cup chicken stock
1 pound turkey breast, skinless, boneless and cubed

1 cup cherry tomatoes, halved
A pinch of salt and black pepper
1 tablespoon rosemary, chopped

Directions:
Heat up a pan with the ghee over medium high heat, add the shallots and the meat and brown for 5 minutes. Add the rest of the ingredients, bring to a simmer and cook over medium heat for 25 minutes, stirring often. Divide into bowls and serve.

Nutrition: calories 150, fat 4, fiber 1, carbs 3, protein 10

Turkey and Cabbage Mix

Try it soon! You will make it a second time as well!

Preparation time: 10 minutes
Cooking time: 30 minutes
Servings: 4

Ingredients:
1 red cabbage, shredded
1 pound turkey breast, skinless, boneless and cubed
2 tablespoons olive oil
2 garlic cloves, mined
2 spring onions, chopped
1 cup tomato passata
1 tablespoon cilantro, chopped
A pinch of salt and black pepper

Directions:
Heat up a pan with the oil over medium heat, add the onions and the garlic and sauté for 2 minutes.
Add the meat and brown for 6 minutes more.

Add the rest of the ingredients, toss, bring to a simmer and cook over medium heat for 20 minutes more.

Divide everything into bowls and serve.

Nutrition: calories 240, fat 15, fiber 1, carbs 3, protein 25

Chili Turkey and Broccoli

This great keto dish is perfect for a cold and rainy day!

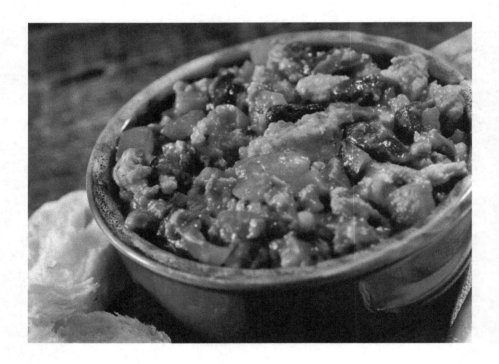

Preparation time: 10 minutes
Cooking time: 30 minutes
Servings: 4

Ingredients:
1 pound turkey breast, skinless, boneless and cubed
1 cup broccoli florets
1 cup chicken stock

2 shallots, chopped

1 tablespoon olive oil

A pinch of salt and black pepper

1 teaspoon chili powder

1 tablespoon chipotle peppers, chopped

½ teaspoon garlic powder

1 tablespoon cilantro, chopped

Directions:

Heat up a pan with the oil over medium heat, add the shallots and the meat and brown for 10 minutes.

Add the stock and the other ingredients except the cilantro, toss, bring to a simmer and cook over medium heat for 20 minutes more.

Add the cilantro, stir, divide into bowls and serve.

Nutrition: calories 154, fat 5, fiber 3, carbs 2, protein 27

Ground Turkey and Bell Peppers

You will make this in no time!

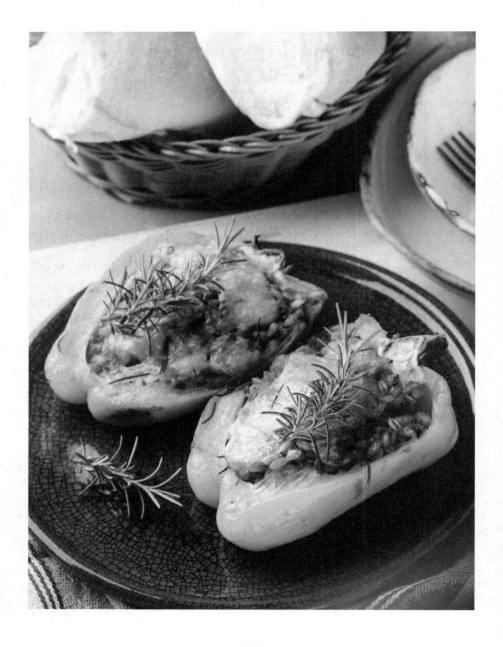

Preparation time: 10 minutes
Cooking time: 30 minutes
Servings: 4

Ingredients:
1 pound turkey meat, ground
1 tablespoon olive oil
3 garlic cloves, minced
1 cup tomatoes, chopped
1 red bell pepper, cut into strips
1 green bell pepper, cut into strips
A pinch of salt and black pepper
1 tablespoon coriander, ground
2 tablespoons ginger, grated
2 tablespoons chili powder

Directions:
Heat up a pan with the oil over medium heat, add the garlic and the meat and brown for 5 minutes.
Add the bell pepper, and cook for 5 minutes more.
Add the rest of the ingredients, toss, bring to a simmer and cook over medium heat for 20 minutes more.
Divide everything into bowls and serve.

Nutrition: calories 240, fat 4, fiber 3, carbs 2, protein 12

Chicken and Walnuts Salad

It's healthy, it's fresh and very delicious!

Preparation time: 10 minutes
Cooking time: 0 minutes
Servings: 4

Ingredients:
2 cups baby arugula
2 cups rotisserie chicken, skinless, boneless and shredded
3 tablespoons walnuts, chopped
2 tablespoons olive oil
2 tablespoon lime juice
A pinch of salt and black pepper
1 tablespoon chives, chopped

Directions:
In a salad bowl, combine the chicken with the walnuts, arugula and the other ingredients, toss and serve.

Nutrition: calories 120, fat 2, fiber 1, carbs 3, protein 7

Ketogenic Meat Recipes

Oregano Pork Chops

This is so yummy and simple to make at home!

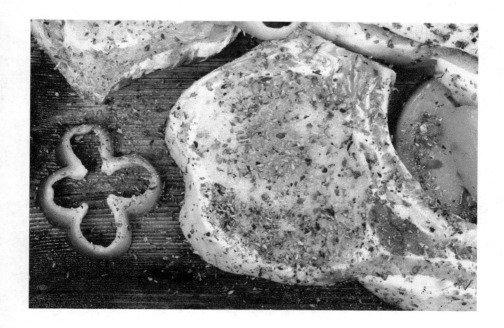

Preparation time: 10 minutes
Cooking time: 36 minutes
Servings: 4

Ingredients:
4 pork chops
1 tablespoon oregano, chopped

2 tablespoons olive oil

1 cup tomato passata

A pinch of salt and black pepper

1 tablespoon cilantro, chopped

2 tablespoons lime juice

Directions:

Heat up a pan with the oil over medium high heat, add the pork chops and the oregano, and brown for 3 minutes on each side.

Add the rest of the ingredients, toss, bring to a simmer and cook over medium heat for 30 minutes.

Divide the mix between plates and serve.

Nutrition: calories 210, fat 10, fiber 2, carbs 6, protein 19

Coconut Beef

These spicy pork chops will impress you for sure!

Preparation time: 10 minutes
Cooking time: 8 hours
Servings: 4

Ingredients:
1 pound beef stew meat, cubed
1 cup beef stock
1 tablespoon coconut oil
1 cup coconut cream
2 shallots, chopped
2 celery ribs, roughly chopped
2 garlic cloves, minced
1 tablespoon chili powder
2 teaspoons cumin, ground
A pinch of salt and black pepper

Directions:
In your slow cooker, combine the meat with the stock and the other ingredients, put the lid on and cook on Low for 8 hours.
Divide everything into bowls and serve.

Nutrition: calories 200, fat 8, fiber 1, carbs 5.3, protein 26

Beef, Tomato and Peppers

It will soon become your favorite keto dinner dish!

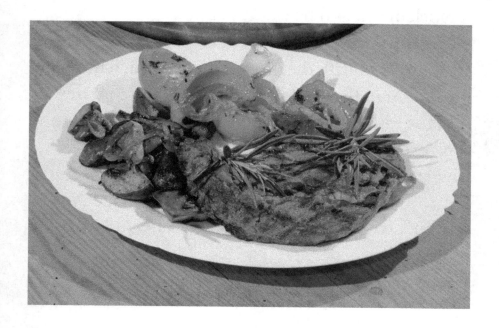

Preparation time: 10 minutes
Cooking time: 35 minutes
Servings: 4

Ingredients:
1 cup beef stock
1 pound beef stew meat, cubed
2 tomatoes, cubed
2 shallots, chopped
1 red bell pepper, cut into strips

1 yellow bell pepper, cut into strips

2 tablespoons olive oil

¼ teaspoon garlic powder

A pinch of salt and black pepper

Directions:

Heat up a pan with the oil over medium high heat, add the meat and the shallots and brown for 5 minutes.

Add the rest of the ingredients, bring to a simmer and cook over medium heat for 30 minutes more.

Divide everything into bowls and serve.

Nutrition: calories 224, fat 15, fiber 1, carbs 3, protein 19

Pork Meatballs

This will be one of the best keto dishes you'll ever try!

Preparation time: 10 minutes
Cooking time: 10 minutes
Servings: 4

Ingredients:
½ cup almond meal
2 eggs
2 pounds pork stew meat, ground
A pinch of salt and black pepper
2 tablespoons cilantro, chopped
2 garlic cloves, minced
2 shallots, chopped
2 tablespoons olive oil

Directions:
In a bowl, mix the pork with the eggs and the other ingredients except the oil, stir well and shape medium meatballs out of this mix.
Heat up a pan with the oil over medium heat, add the meatballs, cook them for 5 minutes on each side, divide between plates and serve with a side salad.

Nutrition: calories 643, fat 37.1, fiber 1.5, carbs 3.3, protein 71.8

Herbed Beef Mix

It's so juicy and delicious!

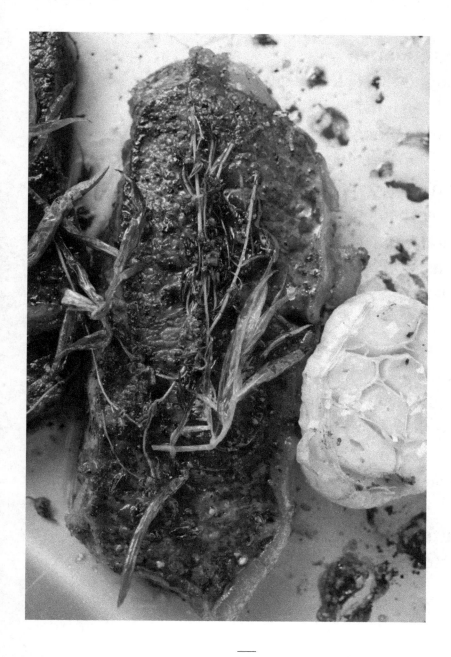

Preparation time: 10 minutes
Cooking time: 30 minutes
Servings: 4

Ingredients:
2 pounds beef stew meat, cubed
2 tablespoons ghee, melted
2 spring onions, chopped
1 cup beef stock
1 tablespoon rosemary, chopped
1 tablespoon parsley, chopped
1 tablespoon tarragon, chopped
1 teaspoon chili powder
½ teaspoon cumin, ground

Directions:
Heat up a pan with the ghee over medium heat, add the meat and spring onions and brown for 5 minutes. Add the rest of the ingredients, toss, bring to a simmer and cook over medium heat for 25 minutes more. Divide everything between plates and serve
.

Nutrition: calories 700, fat 56, fiber 2, carbs 13.10, protein 70

Sage Beef

This looks so good and it tastes wonderful!

Preparation time: 10 minutes
Cooking time: 35 minutes
Servings: 4

Ingredients:
2 garlic cloves, minced
1 pound beef stew meat, cubed
2 tablespoons ghee, melted
2 shallots, chopped
1 celery stalks, chopped
½ cup beef stock
A pinch of salt and black pepper
1 teaspoon cumin, ground
1 tablespoon sage, chopped

Directions:
Heat up a pan with the oil over medium high heat, add the garlic and the shallots and sauté for 5 minutes.
Add the meat and brown for 5 minutes more.
Add the rest of the ingredients, toss, bring to a simmer and cook over medium heat for 25 minutes.

Nutrition: calories 222, fat 10, fiber 2, carbs 8, protein 21

Beef Casserole

This is so special and of course, it's 100% keto!

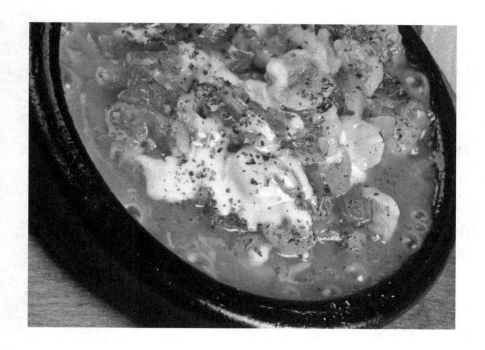

Preparation time: 10 minutes
Cooking time: 35 minutes
Servings: 6

Ingredients:
1 pound beef stew meat, ground
¼ cup beef stock
2 shallots, chopped
2 tablespoons avocado oil

A pinch of salt and black pepper

½ teaspoon red pepper flakes, crushed

A pinch of cayenne pepper

1 cup cherry tomatoes, halved

1 cup zucchinis, cubed

1 cup parmesan, grated

1 tablespoon chives, chopped

Directions:

Heat up a pan with the oil over medium heat, add the meat and shallots and brown for 5 minutes.

Add the tomatoes and the other ingredients except the parmesan and the chives, toss and cook for 5 minutes more.

Sprinkle the cheese and chives on top, introduce the pan in the oven, bake at 375 degrees F for 25 minutes, divide between plates and serve hot.

Nutrition: calories 456, fat 35, fiber 3, carbs 4, protein 32

Thyme Beef and Leeks

It's always amazing to discover such interesting dishes!

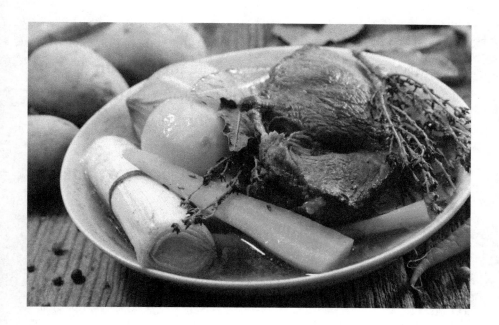

Preparation time: 10 minutes
Cooking time: 35 minutes
Servings: 4

Ingredients:
2 pounds beef stew meat, cubed
2 tablespoons ghee, melted
A pinch of salt and black pepper
2 leeks, sliced

1 cup beef stock

3 garlic cloves, minced

1 teaspoon oregano, dried

1 tablespoon thyme, chopped

Directions:

Heat up a pan with the ghee over medium high heat, add the leeks and garlic and sauté for 5 minutes.

Add the meat and brown for 5 minutes more.

Add the stock and the rest of the ingredients, bring to a simmer and cook over medium heat for 25 minutes more.

Divide everything into bowls and serve.

Nutrition: calories 260, fat 7, fiber 2, carbs 4, protein 10

Coconut Pork and Celery

This is so delightful! You've got to try this really soon!

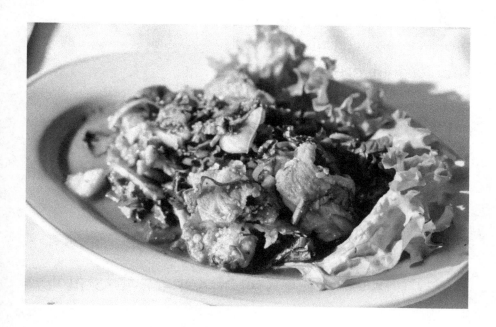

Preparation time: 10 minutes
Cooking time: 8 hours
Servings: 4

Ingredients:
2 shallots, chopped
2 pounds beef stew meat, cubed
1 tablespoon ghee, melted
1 cup tomato passata
2 jalapenos, minced

3 celery ribs, chopped

2 tablespoons coconut aminos

A pinch of salt and black pepper

A pinch of cayenne pepper

2 tablespoons cumin, ground

1 tablespoon oregano, chopped

Directions:

In your slow cooker, combine the meat with the shallots and the other ingredients, put the lid on and cook on Low for 8 hours.

Divide everything between plates and serve.

Nutrition: calories 137, fat 6, fiber 2, carbs 5, protein 17

Pork and Mushroom Meatloaf

This will guarantee your success!

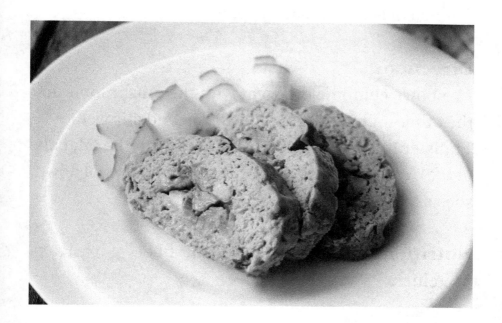

Preparation time: 10 minutes
Cooking time: 50 minutes
Servings: 4

Ingredients:
2 pounds beef stew meat, ground
½ pound white mushrooms, sliced
2 eggs, whisked
1 tablespoon olive oil
2 tablespoons parsley, chopped

2 garlic cloves, minced

½ cup coconut flour

½ cup mozzarella shredded

A pinch of salt and black pepper

Directions:

In a bowl, combine the meat with the mushrooms and the other ingredients except the oil, and stir well. Transfer this into a loaf pan greased with the oil, bake in the oven at 375 degrees F for 50 minutes, cool down, slice and serve.

Nutrition: calories 264, fat 14, fiber 3, carbs 5, protein 24

Minty Beef

You need to make sure there's enough for everyone!

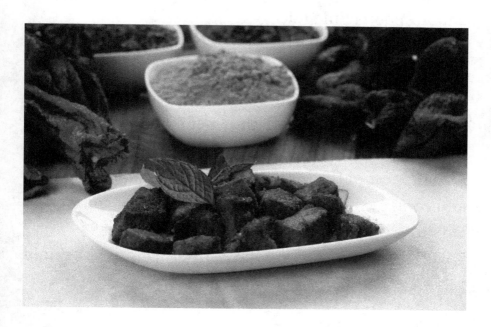

Preparation time: 10 minutes
Cooking time: 30 minutes
Servings: 4

Ingredients:
1 pound beef stew meat, cubed
2 tablespoons ghee, melted
2 shallots, chopped
1 cup beef stock
¼ cup mint, chopped

¼ cup parsley, chopped

A pinch of salt and black pepper

2 garlic cloves, minced

2 tablespoons lime juice

Directions:

Heat up a pan with the ghee over medium heat, add the shallots, garlic and the meat and brown for 5 minutes.

Add the rest of the ingredients, toss, bring to a simmer and cook over medium heat for 25 minutes more.

Divide everything into bowls and serve.

Nutrition: calories 200, fat 4, fiber 1, carbs 3, protein 7

Parsley Pork and Beef Meatballs

A friendly meal can turn into a feast with this keto dish!

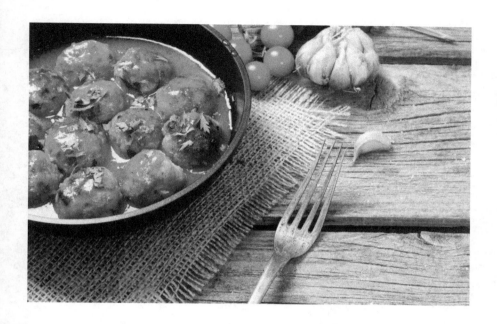

Preparation time: 10 minutes
Cooking time: 12 minutes
Servings: 4

Ingredients:

1 pound beef meat, ground

½ pound pork stew meat, ground

2 eggs, whisked

¼ cup coconut flour

1 cup parsley, minced

2 garlic cloves, minced

2 tablespoons ghee, melted

A pinch of salt and black pepper

Directions:

In a bowl, combine the beef and pork meat with the other ingredients except the ghee, stir well and shape medium meatballs out of this mix.

Heat up a pan with the ghee over medium heat, add the meatballs, cook them for 6 minutes on each side, divide between plates and serve.

Nutrition: calories 435, fat 23, fiber 4, carbs 6, protein 32

Beef with Kale and Leeks

This is so tasty!

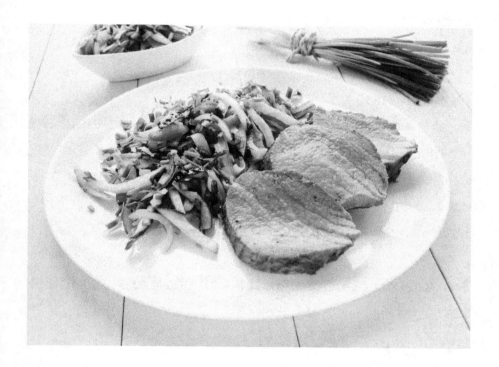

Preparation time: 10 minutes
Cooking time: 30 minutes
Servings: 4

Ingredients:
2 tablespoons olive oil
1 pound beef stew meat, cubed
1 cup kale, torn
2 leeks, chopped

1 cup tomato passata

A pinch of salt and black pepper

1 tablespoon cilantro, chopped

1 teaspoon sweet paprika

½ teaspoon rosemary, dried

Directions:

Heat up a pan with the oil over medium heat, add the leeks and the meat and brown for 5 minutes.

Add the rest of the ingredients, bring to a simmer and cook over medium heat for 25 minutes more.

Divide everything into bowls and serve.

Nutrition: calories 250, fat 5, fiber 1, carbs 3, protein 12

Sesame Beef

A friendly and casual meal requires such a keto dish!

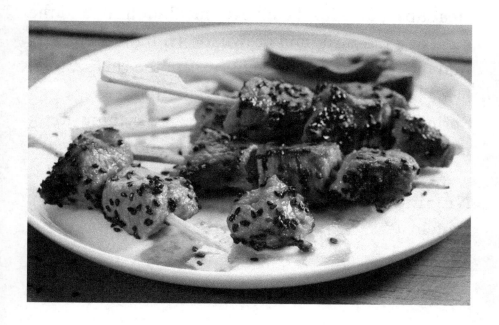

Preparation time: 10 minutes
Cooking time: 35 minutes
Servings: 4

Ingredients:

2 pounds beef stew meat, cubed

2 tablespoons olive oil

2 garlic cloves, minced

A pinch of salt and black pepper

1 tablespoon sesame seeds

1 cup mozzarella cheese, shredded

½ cup beef stock

Directions:

Heat up a pan with the oil over medium heat, add the meat and the garlic and brown for 5 minutes.

Add the rest of the ingredients except the cheese, toss, bring to a simmer and cook for 25 minutes.

Sprinkle the cheese on top, cook everything for 5 minutes more, divide between plates and serve.

Nutrition: calories 554, fat 51, fiber 3, carbs 5, protein 45

Marjoram Beef

It only takes a few minutes to make this special keto recipe!

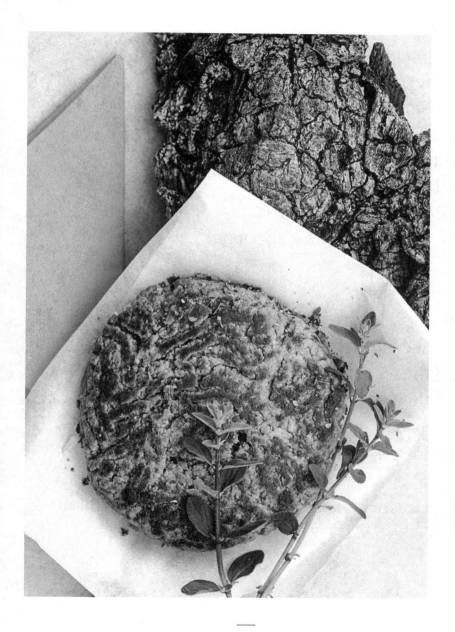

Preparation time: 10 minutes
Cooking time: 30 minutes
Servings: 4

Ingredients:
1 pound beef stew meat, cubed
2 tablespoons ghee, melted
1 red onion, chopped
2 garlic cloves, minced
1 cup beef stock
2 teaspoons sweet paprika
1 tablespoon marjoram, chopped
A pinch of salt and black pepper

Directions:
Heat up a pan with the ghee over medium heat, add the onion and the garlic and sauté for 5 minutes.
Add the meat and brown for 5 minutes more.
Add the rest of the ingredients, bring to a simmer and cook over medium heat for 20 minutes more.
Divide everything into bowls and serve.

Nutrition: calories 320, fat 13, fiber 4, carbs 12, protein 40

Ketogenic Vegetable Recipes

Broccoli Cream

This is so textured and delicious!

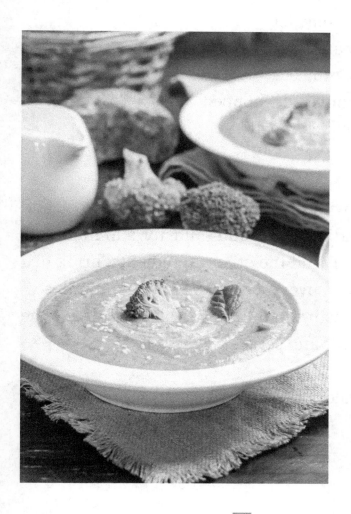

Preparation time: 10 minutes
Cooking time: 20 minutes
Servings: 4

Ingredients:
1 pound broccoli florets
4 cups vegetable stock
2 shallots, chopped
1 teaspoon chili powder
A pinch of salt and black pepper
2 garlic cloves, minced
2 tablespoons olive oil, chopped
1 tablespoon dill, chopped

Directions:
Heat up a pot with the oil over medium high heat, add the shallots and the garlic and sauté for 2 minutes. Add the broccoli and the other ingredients, bring to a simmer and cook over medium heat for 18 minutes. Blend the mix using an immersion blender, divide the cream into bowls and serve.

Nutrition: calories 111, fat 8, fiber 3.3, carbs 10.2, protein 3.7

Cauliflower and Tomatoes Mix

This veggie mix is just delicious!

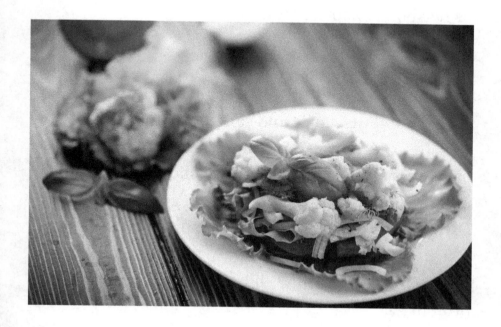

Preparation time: 10 minutes
Cooking time: 30 minutes
Servings: 4

Ingredients:
1 pound cauliflower florets
½ pound cherry tomatoes, halved
2 tablespoons avocado oil
2 shallots, chopped
2 garlic cloves, minced

A pinch of salt and black pepper

1 cup vegetable stock

1 tablespoon coriander, chopped

½ teaspoon allspice, ground

Directions:

Heat up a pan with the oil over medium heat, add the shallots and the garlic and sauté for 2 minutes.

Add the cauliflower and the other ingredients, toss, bring to a simmer and cook over medium heat for 28 minutes more.

Divide everything between plates and serve.

Nutrition: calories 57, fat 1.7, fiber 3.9, carbs 10.7, protein 3.1

Shallots and Kale Soup

A keto soup sounds pretty amazing, doesn't it?

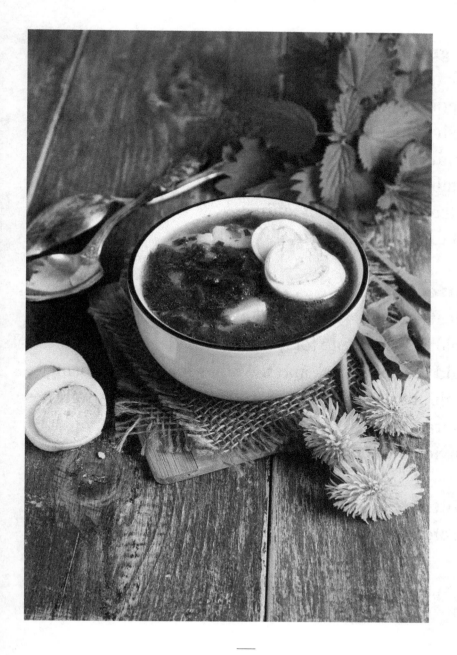

Preparation time: 10 minutes
Cooking time: 20 minutes
Servings: 4

Ingredients:
4 cups chicken stock
1 pound kale, torn
2 shallots, chopped
A pinch of salt and black pepper
1 tablespoon olive oil
2 teaspoons coconut aminos
1 tablespoon cilantro, chopped

Directions:
Heat up a pot with the oil over medium heat, add the shallots and sauté for 5 minutes.
Add the kale, stock and the other ingredients, bring to a simmer and cook over medium heat for 15 minutes more.
Divide the soup into bowls and serve.

Nutrition: calories 98, fat 4.1, fiber 1.7, carbs 13.1, protein 4.1

Hot Kale Pan

You can even have this for dinner!

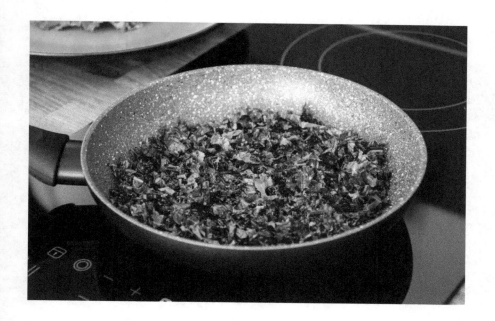

Preparation time: 10 minutes
Cooking time: 23 minutes
Servings: 4

Ingredients:

1 red onion, chopped
1 pound kale, roughly torn
1 cup baby bella mushrooms, halved
A pinch of salt and black pepper
1 tablespoon olive oil

3 garlic cloves, minced

½ teaspoon hot paprika

½ tablespoon red pepper flakes, crushed

1 tablespoon dill, chopped

3 tablespoons coconut aminos

Directions:

Heat up a pan with the oil over medium heat, add the onion and the garlic and sauté for 5 minutes.

Add the mushrooms, and sauté them for 3 minutes more.

Add the kale and the other ingredients, toss, cook over medium heat for 15 minutes more, divide into bowls and serve.

Nutrition: calories 100, fat 3, fiber 1, carbs 2, protein 6

Baked Broccoli

It's simple, it's easy and very delicious!

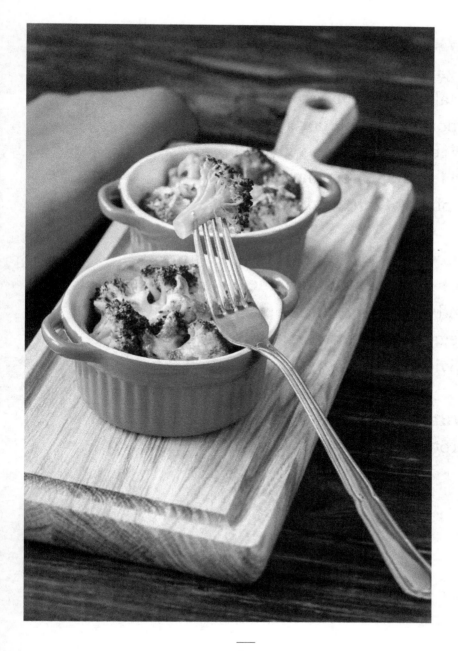

Preparation time: 10 minutes
Cooking time: 20 minutes
Servings: 4

Ingredients:
2 garlic cloves, minced
2 tablespoons olive oil
1 pound broccoli florets
½ teaspoon nutmeg, ground
½ teaspoons rosemary, dried
A pinch of salt and black pepper

Directions:
In a roasting pan, combine the broccoli with the garlic and the other ingredients, toss and bake at 400 degrees F for 20 minutes.
Divide the mix between plates and serve.

Nutrition: calories 150, fat 4.1, fiber 1, carbs 3.2, protein 2

Leeks Cream

This will impress you!

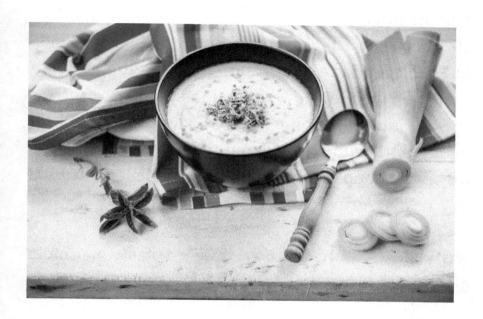

Preparation time: 10 minutes
Cooking time: 30 minutes
Servings: 4

Ingredients:
4 leeks, sliced
4 cups vegetable stock
1 tablespoon olive oil
2 shallots, chopped
1 tablespoon rosemary, chopped
A pinch of salt and black pepper

1 cup heavy cream
1 tablespoon chives, chopped

Directions:
Heat up a pot with the oil over medium high heat, add the shallots and the leeks and sauté for 5 minutes.
Add the stock and the other ingredients except the chives, bring to a simmer and cook over medium heat for 25 minutes stirring from time to time.
Blend the soup using an immersion blender, ladle it into bowls, sprinkle the chives on top and serve.

Nutrition: calories 150, fat 3, fiber 1, carbs 2, protein 6

Fennel Soup

It's so delightful and delicious! Try it!

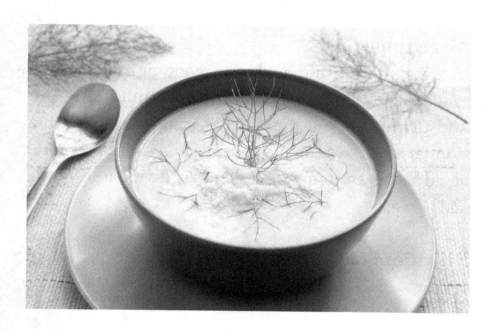

Preparation time: 10 minutes
Cooking time: 25 minutes
Servings: 4

Ingredients:
2 fennel bulb, sliced
2 tablespoons olive oil
2 shallots, chopped
3 garlic cloves, minced
4 cups chicken stock

A pinch of salt and black pepper
1 cup heavy cream
1 tablespoon dill, chopped

Directions:
Heat up a pot with the oil over medium heat, add the shallots and the garlic and sauté for 5 minutes.
Add the fennel and the other ingredients, bring to a simmer, cook over medium heat for 20 minutes more, blend using an immersion blender, divide into bowls and serve.

Nutrition: calories 140, fat 2, fiber 1, carbs 5, protein 10

Cauliflower and Green Beans

This Iranian style keto stew is so tasty and easy to make!

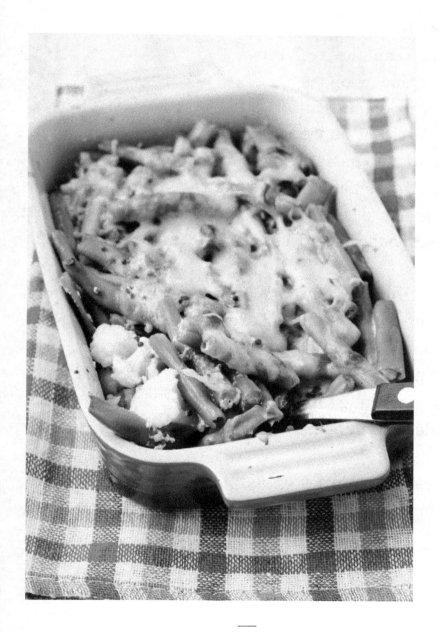

Preparation time: 10 minutes
Cooking time: 30 minutes
Servings: 4

Ingredients:
1 pound cauliflower florets
1 red onion, chopped
1 tablespoon olive oil
2 garlic cloves minced
1 cup tomato passata
A pinch of salt and black pepper
½ pound green beans, trimmed and halved
1 tablespoon cilantro, chopped

Directions:
Heat up a pot with the oil over medium high heat, add the onion and the garlic and sauté for 5 minutes.
Add the cauliflower and the other ingredients, toss and cook everything for 25 minutes more.
Divide everything between plates and serve.

Nutrition: calories 93, fat 3.7, fiber 5.9, carbs 13.7, protein 4.1

Bok Choy Soup

It's a textured and creamy keto mix you have to try soon!

Preparation time: 10 minutes
Cooking time: 25 minutes
Servings: 4

Ingredients:
2 tablespoons coconut oil, melted
1 pound bok choy, torn
2 shallots, chopped
4 cups chicken stock
1 cup heavy cream
1 tablespoon cilantro, chopped
A pinch of salt and black pepper
½ teaspoon nutmeg, ground

Directions:
Heat up a pot with the oil over medium heat, add the shallots and sauté for 5 minutes.

Add the bok choy and the other ingredients, bring to a simmer and cook over medium heat for 20 minutes.

Blend the soup using an immersion blender, divide into bowls and serve.

Nutrition: calories 192, fat 18.8, fiber 1.2, carbs 5.1, protein 3.2

Cabbage Sauté

This is so tasty!

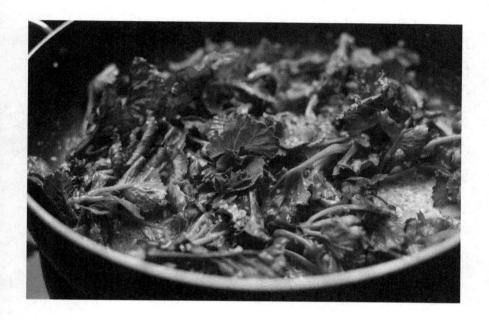

Preparation time: 10 minutes
Cooking time: 20 minutes
Servings: 4

Ingredients:

2 garlic cloves, minced

2 shallots, chopped

1 tablespoon olive oil

1 green cabbage head, shredded

1 cup tomatoes, cubed

1 teaspoon lime juice

A pinch of salt and black pepper

1 tablespoon cilantro, chopped

Directions:

Heat up a pan with the oil over medium high heat, add the shallots and the garlic and sauté for 5 minutes.

Add the cabbage and the other ingredients, toss and cook over medium heat for 15 minutes more.

Divide everything between plates and serve.

Nutrition: calories 89, fat 3.8, fiber 5.1, carbs 13.5, protein 2.9

Mustard Greens Sauté

This tasty dish will be ready in not time!

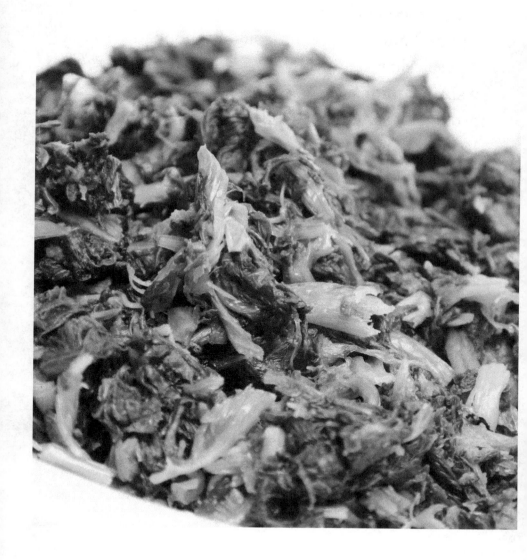

Preparation time: 10 minutes
Cooking time: 20 minutes
Servings: 4

Ingredients:
1 tablespoon olive oil
1 pound mustard greens, roughly chopped
2 garlic cloves, minced
2 spring onions, chopped
A pinch of salt and black pepper
½ cup chicken stock
1 tablespoon balsamic vinegar
1 tablespoon cilantro, chopped

Directions:
Heat up a pan with the oil over medium heat, add the garlic and the spring onions, stir and sauté for 5 minutes.
Add the mustard greens and the other ingredients, bring to a simmer and cook over medium heat for 15 minutes more.
Divide everything between plates and serve.

Nutrition: calories 150, fat 12, fiber 2, carbs 4, protein 8

Bok Choy and Tomatoes

This is just fantastic!

Preparation time: 10 minutes
Cooking time: 20 minutes
Servings: 4

Ingredients:
1 pound bok choy
2 shallots, chopped
1 tablespoon olive oil
2 cups tomatoes, cubed
1 tablespoon balsamic vinegar
½ cup vegetable stock
A pinch of salt and black pepper
1 teaspoon rosemary, dried
1 teaspoon fennel powder
1 tablespoon chives, chopped

Directions:
Heat up a pan with the oil over medium heat, add the shallots and sauté for 3 minutes.

Add the bok choy and the other ingredients, bring to a simmer and cook over heat for 17 minutes.

Divide the mix between plates and serve

Nutrition: calories 120, fat 8, fiber 1, carbs 3, protein 7

Sesame Savoy Cabbage

Everyone can make this simple keto dish! You'll see!

Preparation time: 5 minutes
Cooking time: 20 minutes
Servings: 4

Ingredients:
2 garlic cloves, minced
2 spring onions, chopped
1 Savoy cabbage, shredded
1 tablespoon olive oil
½ cup tomato passata
1 tablespoon sesame seeds

Directions:
Heat up a pan with the oil over medium heat, add the spring onions and the garlic and sauté for 5 minutes. Add the cabbage and the rest of the ingredients, toss, cook over medium heat for 15 minutes more, divide between plates and serve.

Nutrition: calories 120, fat 3, fiber 1, carbs 3, protein 6

Chili Collard Greens

This will really make everyone love your cooking!

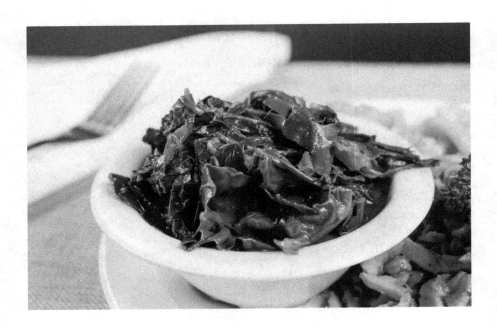

Preparation time: 10 minutes
Cooking time: 20 minutes
Servings: 4

Ingredients:
1 tablespoon chili powder
1 bunch collard greens, roughly chopped
1 tablespoon olive oil
½ cup chicken stock
2 shallots, chopped

1 teaspoon hot paprika

½ teaspoon cumin, ground

A pinch of salt and black pepper

1 tablespoon lime juice

Directions:

Heat up a pan with the oil over medium high heat, add the shallots and sauté for 5 minutes.

Add the collard greens and the other ingredients, toss and cook over medium heat for 15 minutes more.

Divide everything between plates and serve.

Nutrition: calories 245, fat 20, fiber 1, carbs 5, protein 12

Artichokes Soup

This is a keto soup even vegetarians will love!

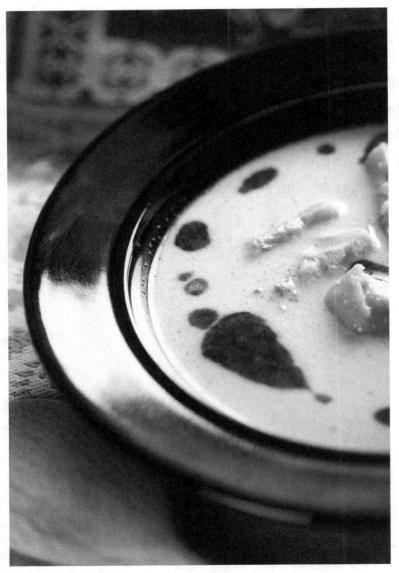

Preparation time: 10 minutes

Cooking time: 35 minutes
Servings: 6

Ingredients:
1 tablespoon olive oil
2 shallots, chopped
10 ounces canned artichokes, drained and quartered
4 cups chicken stock
1 teaspoon smoked paprika
1 teaspoon cumin, ground
A pinch of red pepper flakes
3 celery stalks, chopped
2 tomatoes, cubed
2 tablespoons lime juice
A pinch of salt and black pepper

Directions:
Heat up a pot with the oil over medium high heat, add the shallots and sauté for 5 minutes.
Add the artichokes and the other ingredients, bring to a simmer and cook over medium heat for 30 minutes more.
Ladle the soup into bowls and serve.

Nutrition: calories 150, fat 3, fiber 2, carbs 4, protein 8

Ketogenic Dessert Recipes

Chocolate Pudding

These is so wonderful and delicious!

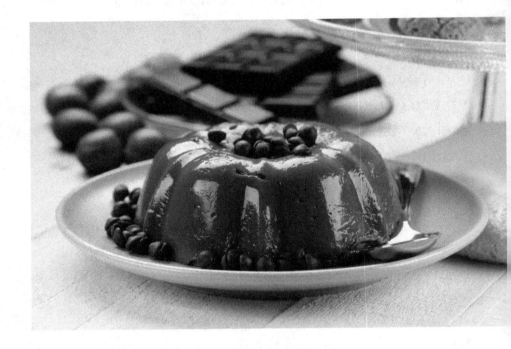

Preparation time: 10 minutes
Cooking time: 20 minutes
Servings: 4

Ingredients:
2 tablespoons cocoa powder

2 tablespoons ghee, melted

2/3 cup heavy cream

2 tablespoons swerve

¼ teaspoon vanilla extract

Directions:

In a bowl, combine the cocoa with the ghee and the other ingredients whisk well and divide into 4 ramekins.

Bake at 350 degrees F for 20 minutes and serve warm.

Nutrition: calories 134, fat 14.1, fiber 0.8, carbs 3.1, protein 0.9

Coffee Cream

This looks and tastes wonderful!

Preparation time: 10 minutes
Cooking time: 15 minutes
Servings: 4

Ingredients:
¼ cup brewed coffee
2 tablespoons swerve
2 cups heavy cream
1 teaspoon vanilla extract
2 tablespoons ghee, melted
2 eggs

Directions:
In a bowl, mix the coffee with the cream and the other ingredients, whisk well and divide into 4 ramekins and whisk well.
Introduce the ramekins in the oven at 350 degrees F and bake for 15 minutes.
Serve warm.

Nutrition: calories 300, fat 30.8, fiber 0, carbs 3, protein 4

Walnut Balls

You must try these today!

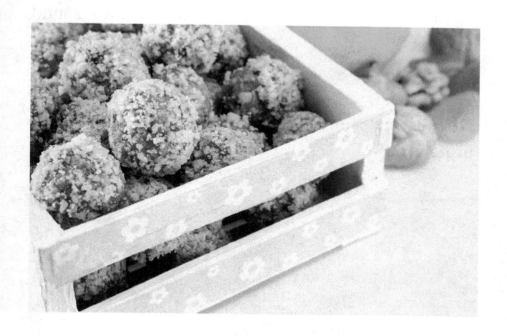

Preparation time: 10 minutes
Cooking time: 0 minutes
Servings: 6

Ingredients:
½ cup ghee, melted
4 tablespoons walnuts, chopped
1 tablespoon stevia
¼ cup coconut flesh, unsweetened and shredded

Directions:

In a bowl, combine the walnuts with the ghee and the other ingredients, stir well and spoon into round moulds.

Keep in the fridge until you serve them.

Nutrition: calories 194, fat 21.2, fiber 0.7, carbs 1, protein 1.4

Vanilla Cream

It's more than you can imagine!

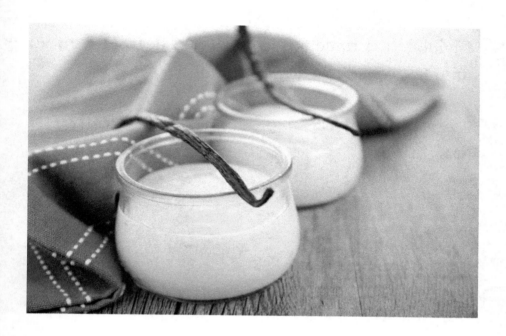

Preparation time: 10 minutes
Cooking time: 20 minutes
Servings: 4

Ingredients:
2 cups heavy cream
2 tablespoons stevia
1 teaspoon vanilla extract
1 cup heavy cream
2 eggs, whisked

1 teaspoon baking powder

Directions:

In a bowl, combine the cream with the stevia and the other ingredients and whisk well.

Divide into 4 ramekins, cook at 390 degrees F for 20 minutes, cool down and serve.

Nutrition: calories 346, fat 35.5, fiber 0, carbs 3.4, protein 4.6

Berry Cream

It's so delicious!

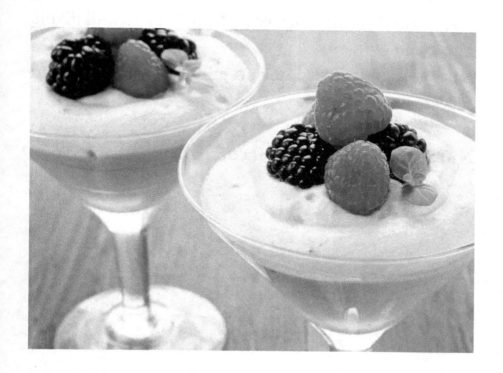

Preparation time: 10 minutes
Cooking time: 20 minutes
Servings: 4
Ingredients:
1 cup cream cheese
2 cups blackberries
1 tablespoon lime juice
1 tablespoon swerve
½ cup heavy cream

Directions:

In your blender, combine the blackberries with the cream and the other ingredients, pulse well and divide into 4 ramekins.

Bake at 350 degrees F for 20 minutes, cool down and serve.

Nutrition: calories 289, fat 26.1, fiber 3.9, carbs 10.3, protein 5.7

Cream Cheese Ramekins

This special dessert will impress your loved ones for sure!

Preparation time: 10 minutes
Cooking time: 15 minutes
Servings: 6

Ingredients:
1 tablespoon vanilla extract
3 tablespoons ghee, melted
16 ounces cream cheese
½ cup swerve
1 teaspoon vanilla extract

Directions:
In a bowl, combine the vanilla with the ghee and the other ingredients, whisk well, divide into 6 ramekins, bake at 350 degrees F for 15 minutes, cool down and serve.

Nutrition: calories 329, fat 32.7, fiber 0, carbs 2.5, protein 5.7

Avocado Cream

This is a keto friendly dessert idea you must try!

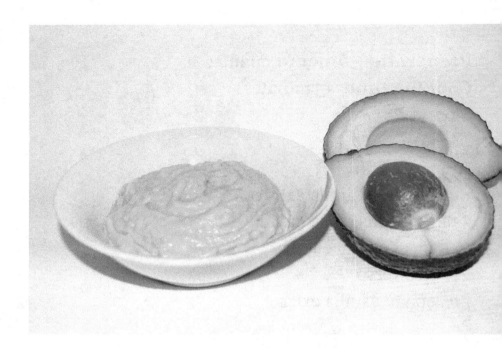

Preparation time: 10 minutes
Cooking time: 15 minutes
Servings: 4

Ingredients:
2 tablespoons avocado oil
8 ounces cream cheese
2 avocados, peeled, pitted and mashed
2 eggs, whisked

1 teaspoon baking powder

½ cup swerve

Directions:

In your blender, combine the cream cheese with the avocados and the other ingredients, pulse well, divide into 4 ramekins and bake at 360 degrees F for 15 minutes.

Cool the cream down and serve.

Nutrition: calories 312, fat 29.5, fiber 3.3, carbs 16.7, protein 8

Strawberry Stew

This is easy to make!

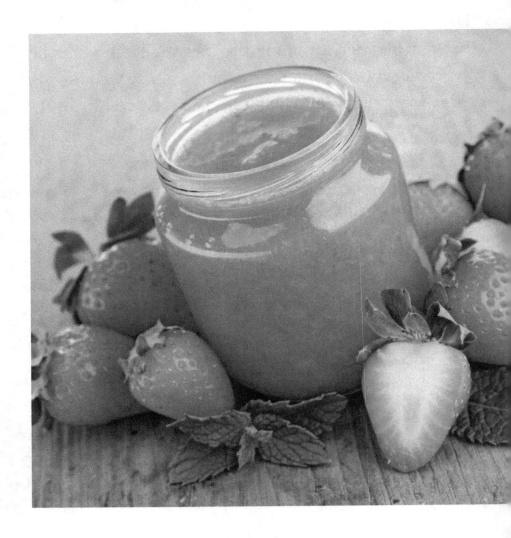

Preparation time: 10 minutes
Cooking time: 15 minutes
Servings: 4

Ingredients:

½ cup swerve

1 pound strawberries, halved

2 cups water

1 teaspoon vanilla extract

Directions:

In a pan, combine the strawberries with the swerve and the other ingredients, toss gently, bring to a simmer and cook over medium heat for 15 minutes. Divide into bowls and serve cold.

Nutrition: calories 40, fat 4.3, fiber 2.3, carbs 3.4, protein 0.8

Coconut Muffins

Everyone will adore these coconut delights!

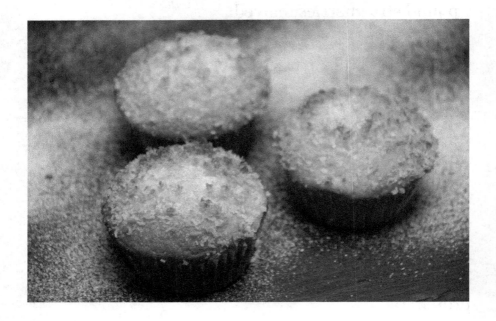

Preparation time: 10 minutes
Cooking time: 25 minutes
Servings: 8

Ingredients:
½ cup ghee, melted
3 tablespoons swerve
1 cup coconut, unsweetened and shredded
¼ cup cocoa powder
2 eggs, whisked

¼ teaspoon vanilla extract

1 teaspoon baking powder

Directions:

In bowl, combine the ghee with the swerve, coconut and the other ingredients, stir well and divide into a lined muffin pan.

Bake at 370 degrees F for 25 minutes, cool down and serve.

Nutrition: calories 344, fat 35.1, fiber 3.4, carbs 8.3, protein 4.5

Blueberries Mousse

This is just hypnotizing! It's great!

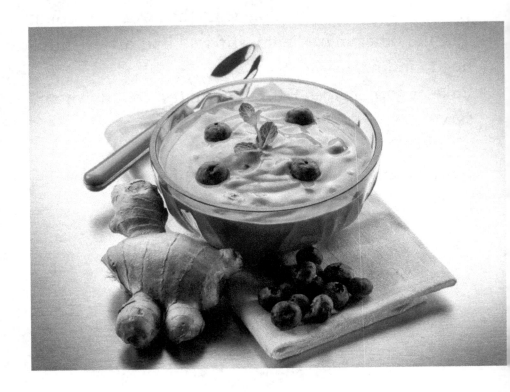

Preparation time: 10 minutes
Cooking time: 0 minutes
Servings: 6

Ingredients:

8 ounces heavy cream
1 teaspoon vanilla extract
1 tablespoon stevia

1 cup blueberries

Directions:

In a blender, combine the cream with the other ingredients, pulse well, divide into bowls and serve cold.

Nutrition: calories 219, fat 21.1, fiber 0.9, carbs 7, protein

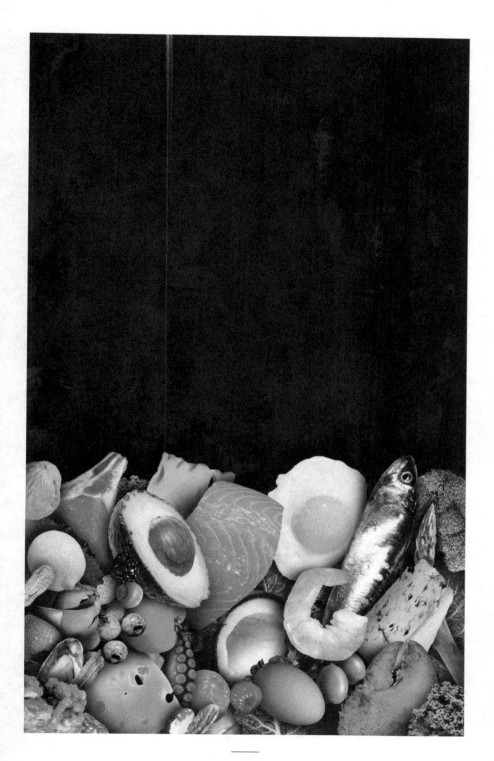

RECIPE INDEX

A

Artichokes Soup 86

Avocado Cream 98

B

Baked Broccoli 67

Beef Casserole 41

Beef with Kale and Leeks 53

Beef, Tomato and Peppers 33

Berry Cream 95

Blueberries Mousse 104

Bok Choy and Tomatoes 81

Bok Choy Soup 75

Broccoli Cream 59

C

Cabbage Sauté 77

Cauliflower and Green Beans 73

Cauliflower and Tomatoes Mix 61

Chicken and Raspberries Salad 16

Chicken and Salsa 10

Chicken and Walnuts Salad 28

Chili Collard Greens 84

Chili Turkey and Broccoli 24

Chocolate Pudding 88

Coconut Beef 31

Coconut Muffins 102

Coconut Pork and Celery 45

Coffee Cream 90

Cream Cheese Ramekins 97

Creamy Turkey 12

D

Duck and Zucchinis 14

F

Fennel Soup 71

G

Ground Turkey and Bell Peppers 26

H

Herbed Beef Mix 37

Hot Kale Pan 65

L

Leeks Cream 69

M

Marjoram Beef 57

Minty Beef 49

Mustard Greens Sauté 79

O

Oregano Pork Chops 29

P

Parsley Pork and Beef Meatballs 51

Pork and Mushroom Meatloaf 47

Pork Meatballs 35

S

Sage Beef 39

Sesame Beef 55

Sesame Savoy Cabbage 83

Shallots and Kale Soup 63

Strawberry Stew 100

T

Thyme Beef and Leeks 43

Turkey and Cabbage Mix 22

Turkey and Spinach 18

Turkey and Tomatoes 20

V

Vanilla Cream 93

W

Walnut Balls 91

MEASUREMENTS & CONVERSIONS

	US STANDARD	US STANDARD (OUNCES)	METRIC (APPROXIMATE)
VOLUME EQUIVALENTS (LIQUID)	2 tablespoon	1 fl. oz.	30 mL
	1/4 cup	2 fl. oz.	60 mL
	1/2 cup	4 fl. oz.	120 mL
	1 cup	8 fl. oz.	240 mL
	1 1/2 cup	12 fl. oz.	355 mL
	2 cups or 1 pint	16 fl. oz.	475 mL
VOLUME EQUIVALENTS DRY	1/4 teaspoon		1 mL
	1/2 teaspoon		2 mL
	1 teaspoon		5 mL
	1 tablespoon		15 mL
	1/4 cup		59 mL
	1/3 cup		79 mL
	1/2 cup		118 mL
	2/3 cup		156 mL
	3/4 cup		177 mL
	1 cup		235 mL
	2 cups or 1 pint		475 mL
	3 cup		700 mL
	4 cups or 1 quart		1 L
WEIGHT EQUIVALENTS	1/2 ounce		15 g
	1 ounce		30 g
	2 ounces		60 g
	4 ounces		115 g
	8 ounces		225 g
	12 ounces		340 g
	16 ounces or 1 pound		455 g

	FAHRENHEIT (F)	CELSIUS (C) (APPROXIMATE)
OVEN TEMPERATURES	250 °F	120 °C
	300 °F	150 °C
	325 °F	180 °C
	375 °F	190 °C
	400 °F	200 °C
	425 °F	220 °C
	450 °F	230 °C

CPSIA information can be obtained
at www.ICGtesting.com
Printed in the USA
BVHW011530250621
610444BV00010B/180